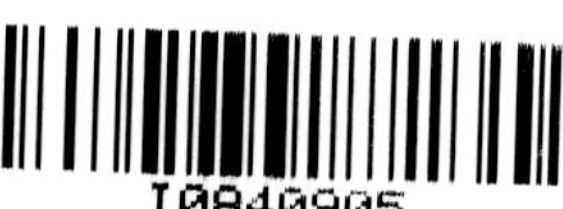

THIS NOTEBOOK BELONGS TO:

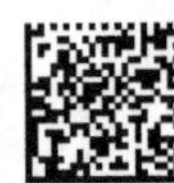